Wealthy Lotus

https://wealthylotus.com

Copyright © All rights reserved.

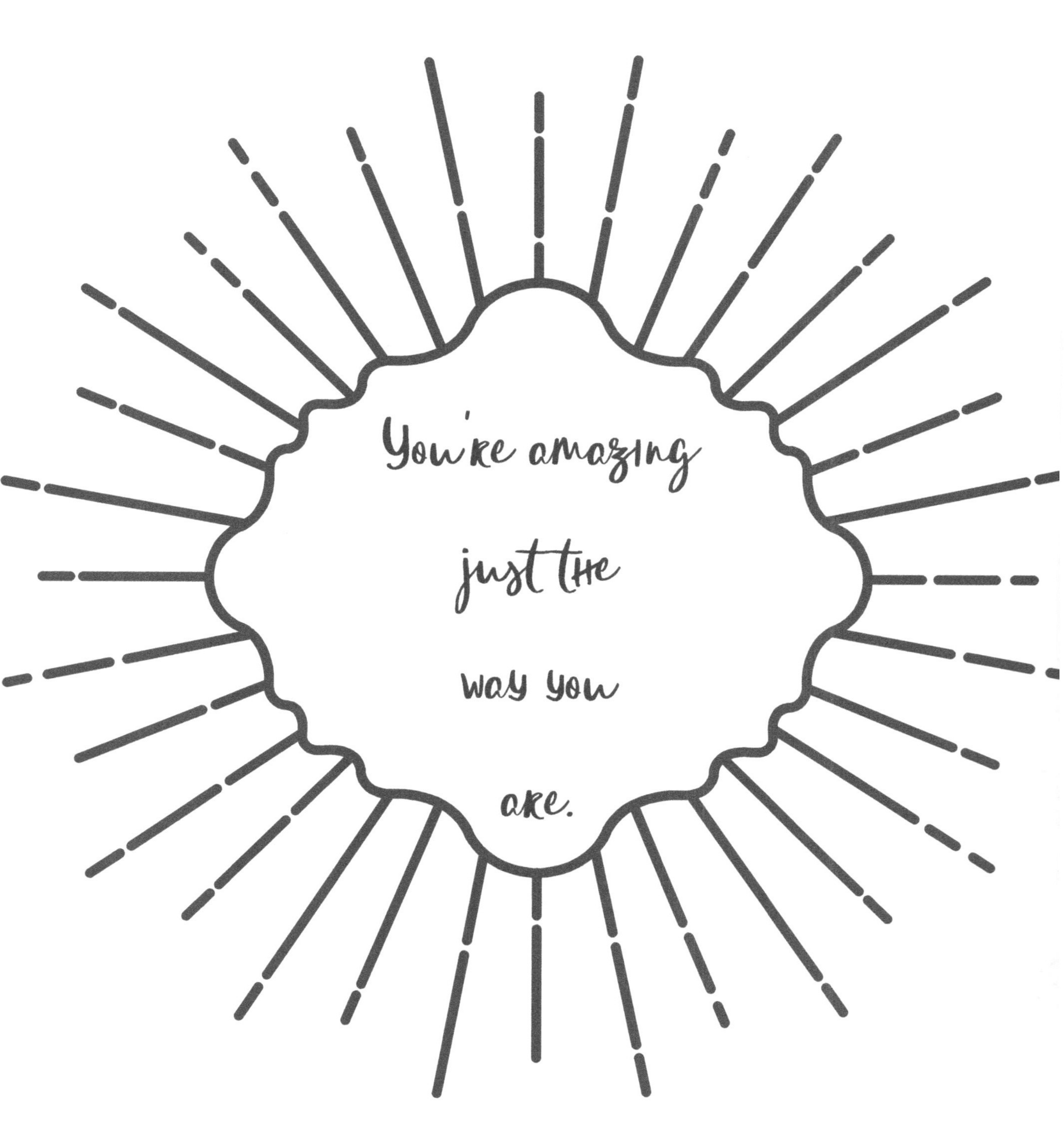

You're amazing
just the
way you
are.

www.ingramcontent.com/pod-procuct-compliance
Lightning Source LLC
Chambersburg PA
CBHW080027260726
48658CB00007B/2500